Lessons Learned on My Commute: Companion Journal

Becoming Your Best Self Blueprint

By Jorge Urquiola

Lessons Learned on My Commute: Companion Journal: Becoming Your Best Self Blueprint

Copyright © 2025 by Jorge Urquiola

All rights reserved. No portion of this book may be reproduced, stored in a retrieval system, or transmitted in any form or by any means—electronic, mechanical, photocopy, recording, scanning, or other—except for brief quotations in critical reviews or articles, without the prior written permission of the publisher.

ISBN 979-8-9999669-4-0

Cover design by: Soledad Ludueña of Luna Design & Jorge Urquiola

Table of Contents

1. Introduction
2. Weekly Habit Tracker
3. Weekly Exercise Tracker
4. Daily Reflection Pages
5. Daily Food Journal
6. Weekly Deep Reflection Prompts
7. Weekly Review Prompts
8. Final Thoughts

Section 1: Introduction

Lessons Learned on My Commute: Companion Journal is your practical, no-fluff workbook for turning intention into daily action. Built around the SHAVE GAMERS habit system, it combines undated weekly and daily pages so you can start anytime and build momentum fast. Inside you'll track keystone habits, log workouts and steps, reflect on what's working, and plan your next three priorities—without losing sight of the bigger "why." Deep-dive prompts (inspired by executive coach Jerry Colonna) help you get honest with yourself, while curated quotes keep you motivated. Pair it with *Lessons Learned on My Commute* or use it solo as your blueprint for becoming your best self—physically, mentally, and emotionally.

What's inside:

- Weekly Habit Tracker using the SHAVE GAMERS framework
- Weekly Fitness Tracker for steps, duration, and workouts
- Daily Reflection pages for gratitude, wins, challenges, and priorities
- Daily Food Journal to build awareness around nutrition and weight trends
- Weekly Review + "Top 3 Goals" to lock in progress and reset with intention
- Deep Reflection Prompts to clarify values, patterns, and next actions
- Inspirational quotes to sustain motivation throughout the journey

Perfect for: high performers, students, entrepreneurs, and anyone who wants a simple, repeatable system to elevate habits and mindset—one week at a time.

Use this workbook as your personal space to cultivate clarity, discipline, and purpose.

"You are under no obligation to be who you were five minutes ago."

– Alan Watts

Weekly Habit Tracker

Track your habits using the **SHAVE GAMERS** framework. Use this weekly template to keep yourself accountable:

Habits:	Monday	Tuesday	Wednesday	Thursday	Friday	Saturday	Sunday
Sleep							
Hydration							
Affirmations							
Visualizations							
Exercise							
Gratitude							
Audible / Learning							
Meditation							
Eat Healthy							
Relationships							
Scribing							

WEEKLY FITNESS TRACKER

Monday	Daily Steps:	Duration:
Workout		

Tuesday	Daily Steps:	Duration:
Workout		

Wednesday	Daily Steps:	Duration:
Workout		

Thursday	Daily Steps:	Duration:
Workout		

Friday	Daily Steps:	Duration:
Workout		

Saturday	Daily Steps:	Duration:
Workout		

Sunday	Daily Steps:	Duration:
Workout		

Daily Journal / Reflection Page

Date: _____

Today I am grateful for:

- _____
- _____
- _____

Important Tasks for Today:

_____
_____
_____

One thing that made me feel proud / happy:

_____

One thing that made me stressed / challenged:

_____

Daily Reflection:

_____
_____
_____
_____
_____
_____
_____
_____

DAILY FOOD JOURNAL

Current Weight:

Breakfast: _____ am

Lunch: _____ pm

Dinner _____ pm

Snacks

Vegetables (Target 30 per week)	Fruit (2-3 Servings per day)	Processed Foods (Avoid / Minimize)

Daily Journal / Reflection Page

Date: _____

Today I am grateful for:

- _____
- _____
- _____

Important Tasks for Today:

_____
_____
_____

One thing that made me feel proud / happy:

_____

One thing that made me stressed / challenged:

_____

Daily Reflection:

_____
_____
_____
_____
_____
_____
_____
_____

DAILY FOOD JOURNAL

Current Weight:

Breakfast: _____ am

Lunch: _____ pm

Dinner _____ pm

Snacks

Vegetables (Target 30 per week)	Fruit (2-3 Servings per day)	Processed Foods (Avoid / Minimize)

Daily Journal / Reflection Page

Date: _____

Today I am grateful for:

- _____
- _____
- _____

Important Tasks for Today:

_____
_____
_____

One thing that made me feel proud / happy:

_____

One thing that made me stressed / challenged:

_____

Daily Reflection:

_____
_____
_____
_____
_____
_____
_____

DAILY FOOD JOURNAL

Current Weight:

Breakfast: _____ am
Lunch: _____ pm
Dinner _____ pm
Snacks

Vegetables (Target 30 per week)	Fruit (2-3 Servings per day)	Processed Foods (Avoid / Minimize)

Daily Journal / Reflection Page

Date: _____

Today I am grateful for:

- _____
- _____
- _____

Important Tasks for Today:

_____
_____
_____

One thing that made me feel proud / happy:

_____

One thing that made me stressed / challenged:

_____

Daily Reflection:

_____
_____
_____
_____
_____
_____
_____
_____

DAILY FOOD JOURNAL

Current Weight: _____

Breakfast: _____ am

Lunch: _____ pm

Dinner _____ pm

Snacks

Vegetables (Target 30 per week)	Fruit (2-3 Servings per day)	Processed Foods (Avoid / Minimize)

Daily Journal / Reflection Page

Date: _____

Today I am grateful for:

- _____
- _____
- _____

Important Tasks for Today:

_____
_____
_____

One thing that made me feel proud / happy:

_____

One thing that made me stressed / challenged:

_____

Daily Reflection:

_____
_____
_____
_____
_____
_____
_____

DAILY FOOD JOURNAL

Current Weight:

Breakfast: _____ am

Lunch: _____ pm

Dinner _____ pm

Snacks

Vegetables (Target 30 per week)	Fruit (2-3 Servings per day)	Processed Foods (Avoid / Minimize)

Daily Journal / Reflection Page

Date: _____

Today I am grateful for:

- _____
- _____
- _____

Important Tasks for Today:

_____
_____
_____

One thing that made me feel proud / happy:

_____

One thing that made me stressed / challenged:

_____

Daily Reflection:

_____
_____
_____
_____
_____
_____
_____
_____

DAILY FOOD JOURNAL

Current Weight:

Breakfast: _____ am

Lunch: _____ pm

Dinner _____ pm

Snacks

Vegetables (Target 30 per week)	Fruit (2-3 Servings per day)	Processed Foods (Avoid / Minimize)

Daily Journal / Reflection Page

Date: _____

Today I am grateful for:

- _____
- _____
- _____

Important Tasks for Today:

_____
_____
_____

One thing that made me feel proud / happy:

_____

One thing that made me stressed / challenged:

_____

Daily Reflection:

_____
_____
_____
_____
_____
_____
_____

DAILY FOOD JOURNAL

Current Weight: _____

Breakfast: _____ am

Lunch: _____ pm

Dinner _____ pm

Snacks

Vegetables (Target 30 per week)	Fruit (2-3 Servings per day)	Processed Foods (Avoid / Minimize)

Deep Reflection Prompts

Use these prompts inspired by Jerry Colonna when you feel the need for deeper introspection:

- How have I been complicit in creating the condition I say I do not want?

- What am I not saying that needs to be said?

- What is being said that I am not hearing?

- Right now, I am feeling…

- In what ways do I deplete myself and run myself into the ground?

- Where am I running from and where am I running to?

Weekly Review Prompts

- What progress have I made this week on my habits?

  _____
  _____

- Where did I feel most energized?

  _____
  _____

- What challenges did I face, and how did I respond?

  _____
  _____

- What could I improve for next week?

  _____
  _____

- Which habit or mindset helped me most?

  _____
  _____

Top 3 Goals for the Coming Week:

1. _____
2. _____
3. _____

"The man who moves a mountain begins by carrying away small stones."

– Confucius

Weekly Habit Tracker

Track your habits using the **SHAVE GAMERS** framework. Use this weekly template to keep yourself accountable:

Habits:	Monday	Tuesday	Wednesday	Thursday	Friday	Saturday	Sunday
Sleep							
Hydration							
Affirmations							
Visualizations							
Exercise							
Gratitude							
Audible / Learning							
Meditation							
Eat Healthy							
Relationships							
Scribing							

WEEKLY FITNESS TRACKER

Monday	Daily Steps:	Duration:
Workout		

Tuesday	Daily Steps:	Duration:
Workout		

Wednesday	Daily Steps:	Duration:
Workout		

Thursday	Daily Steps:	Duration:
Workout		

Friday	Daily Steps:	Duration:
Workout		

Saturday	Daily Steps:	Duration:
Workout		

Sunday	Daily Steps:	Duration:
Workout		

Daily Journal / Reflection Page

Date: _____

Today I am grateful for:

- _____
- _____
- _____

Important Tasks for Today:

_____
_____
_____

One thing that made me feel proud / happy:

_____

One thing that made me stressed / challenged:

_____

Daily Reflection:

_____
_____
_____
_____
_____
_____
_____
_____

DAILY FOOD JOURNAL

Current Weight:

Breakfast: _____ am

Lunch: _____ pm

Dinner _____ pm

Snacks

Vegetables (Target 30 per week)	Fruit (2-3 Servings per day)	Processed Foods (Avoid / Minimize)

Daily Journal / Reflection Page

Date: _____

Today I am grateful for:

- _____
- _____
- _____

Important Tasks for Today:

_____
_____
_____

One thing that made me feel proud / happy:

_____

One thing that made me stressed / challenged:

_____

Daily Reflection:

_____
_____
_____
_____
_____
_____
_____

DAILY FOOD JOURNAL

Current Weight:

Breakfast: _____ am

Lunch: _____ pm

Dinner _____ pm

Snacks

Vegetables (Target 30 per week)	Fruit (2-3 Servings per day)	Processed Foods (Avoid / Minimize)

Daily Journal / Reflection Page

Date: _____

Today I am grateful for:

- _____
- _____
- _____

Important Tasks for Today:

_____
_____
_____

One thing that made me feel proud / happy:

_____

One thing that made me stressed / challenged:

_____

Daily Reflection:

_____
_____
_____
_____
_____
_____
_____
_____

DAILY FOOD JOURNAL

Current Weight: _____

Breakfast: _____ am

Lunch: _____ pm

Dinner _____ pm

Snacks

Vegetables (Target 30 per week)	Fruit (2-3 Servings per day)	Processed Foods (Avoid / Minimize)

Daily Journal / Reflection Page

Date: _____

Today I am grateful for:

- _____
- _____
- _____

Important Tasks for Today:

_____
_____
_____

One thing that made me feel proud / happy:

_____

One thing that made me stressed / challenged:

_____

Daily Reflection:

_____
_____
_____
_____
_____
_____
_____
_____

DAILY FOOD JOURNAL

Current Weight:

Breakfast: _____ am

Lunch: _____ pm

Dinner _____ pm

Snacks

Vegetables (Target 30 per week)	Fruit (2-3 Servings per day)	Processed Foods (Avoid / Minimize)

Daily Journal / Reflection Page

Date: _____

Today I am grateful for:

- _____
- _____
- _____

Important Tasks for Today:

_____
_____
_____

One thing that made me feel proud / happy:

_____

One thing that made me stressed / challenged:

_____

Daily Reflection:

_____
_____
_____
_____
_____
_____
_____

DAILY FOOD JOURNAL

Current Weight:

Breakfast: _____ am

Lunch: _____ pm

Dinner _____ pm

Snacks

Vegetables (Target 30 per week)	Fruit (2-3 Servings per day)	Processed Foods (Avoid / Minimize)

Daily Journal / Reflection Page

Date: _____

Today I am grateful for:

- _____
- _____
- _____

Important Tasks for Today:

_____
_____
_____

One thing that made me feel proud / happy:

_____

One thing that made me stressed / challenged:

_____

Daily Reflection:

_____
_____
_____
_____
_____
_____
_____
_____

DAILY FOOD JOURNAL

Current Weight:

Breakfast: _____ am

Lunch: _____ pm

Dinner _____ pm

Snacks

Vegetables (Target 30 per week)	Fruit (2-3 Servings per day)	Processed Foods (Avoid / Minimize)

Daily Journal / Reflection Page

Date: _____

Today I am grateful for:

- _____
- _____
- _____

Important Tasks for Today:

_____
_____
_____

One thing that made me feel proud / happy:

_____

One thing that made me stressed / challenged:

_____

Daily Reflection:

_____
_____
_____
_____
_____
_____
_____

DAILY FOOD JOURNAL

Current Weight:

Breakfast: _____ am

Lunch: _____ pm

Dinner _____ pm

Snacks

Vegetables (Target 30 per week)	Fruit (2-3 Servings per day)	Processed Foods (Avoid / Minimize)

Deep Reflection Prompts

Use these prompts inspired by Jerry Colonna when you feel the need for deeper introspection:

- How have I been complicit in creating the condition I say I do not want?

- What am I not saying that needs to be said?

- What is being said that I am not hearing?

- Right now, I am feeling…

- In what ways do I deplete myself and run myself into the ground?

- Where am I running from and where am I running to?

Weekly Review Prompts

- What progress have I made this week on my habits?

  _____

  _____

- Where did I feel most energized?

  _____

  _____

- What challenges did I face, and how did I respond?

  _____

  _____

- What could I improve for next week?

  _____

  _____

- Which habit or mindset helped me most?

  _____

  _____

Top 3 Goals for the Coming Week:

1. _____
2. _____
3. _____

"Every action you take is a vote for the type of person you wish to become."

— James Clear

Weekly Habit Tracker

Track your habits using the **SHAVE GAMERS** framework. Use this weekly template to keep yourself accountable:

Habits:	Monday	Tuesday	Wednesday	Thursday	Friday	Saturday	Sunday
Sleep							
Hydration							
Affirmations							
Visualizations							
Exercise							
Gratitude							
Audible / Learning							
Meditation							
Eat Healthy							
Relationships							
Scribing							

WEEKLY FITNESS TRACKER

Monday	Daily Steps:	Duration:
Workout		

Tuesday	Daily Steps:	Duration:
Workout		

Wednesday	Daily Steps:	Duration:
Workout		

Thursday	Daily Steps:	Duration:
Workout		

Friday	Daily Steps:	Duration:
Workout		

Saturday	Daily Steps:	Duration:
Workout		

Sunday	Daily Steps:	Duration:
Workout		

Daily Journal / Reflection Page

Date: _____

Today I am grateful for:

- _____
- _____
- _____

Important Tasks for Today:

_____
_____
_____

One thing that made me feel proud / happy:

_____

One thing that made me stressed / challenged:

_____

Daily Reflection:

_____
_____
_____
_____
_____
_____
_____

DAILY FOOD JOURNAL

Current Weight:

Breakfast: _____ am

Lunch: _____ pm

Dinner _____ pm

Snacks

Vegetables (Target 30 per week)	Fruit (2-3 Servings per day)	Processed Foods (Avoid / Minimize)

Daily Journal / Reflection Page

Date: _____

Today I am grateful for:

- _____
- _____
- _____

Important Tasks for Today:

_____
_____
_____

One thing that made me feel proud / happy:

_____

One thing that made me stressed / challenged:

_____

Daily Reflection:

_____
_____
_____
_____
_____
_____
_____

DAILY FOOD JOURNAL

Current Weight:

Breakfast: _____ am

Lunch: _____ pm

Dinner _____ pm

Snacks

Vegetables (Target 30 per week)	Fruit (2-3 Servings per day)	Processed Foods (Avoid / Minimize)

Daily Journal / Reflection Page

Date: _____

Today I am grateful for:

- _____
- _____
- _____

Important Tasks for Today:

_____
_____
_____

One thing that made me feel proud / happy:

_____

One thing that made me stressed / challenged:

_____

Daily Reflection:

_____
_____
_____
_____
_____
_____
_____

DAILY FOOD JOURNAL

Current Weight:

Breakfast: _____am
Lunch: _____pm
Dinner _____pm
Snacks

Vegetables (Target 30 per week)	Fruit (2-3 Servings per day)	Processed Foods (Avoid / Minimize)

Daily Journal / Reflection Page

Date: _____

Today I am grateful for:

- _____
- _____
- _____

Important Tasks for Today:

_____
_____
_____

One thing that made me feel proud / happy:

_____

One thing that made me stressed / challenged:

_____

Daily Reflection:

_____
_____
_____
_____
_____
_____
_____

DAILY FOOD JOURNAL

Current Weight: _____

Breakfast: _____ am
Lunch: _____ pm
Dinner _____ pm
Snacks

Vegetables (Target 30 per week)	Fruit (2-3 Servings per day)	Processed Foods (Avoid / Minimize)

Daily Journal / Reflection Page

Date: _____

Today I am grateful for:

- _____
- _____
- _____

Important Tasks for Today:

_____
_____
_____

One thing that made me feel proud / happy:

_____

One thing that made me stressed / challenged:

_____

Daily Reflection:

_____
_____
_____
_____
_____
_____
_____

DAILY FOOD JOURNAL

Current Weight:

Breakfast: _____ am

Lunch: _____ pm

Dinner _____ pm

Snacks

Vegetables (Target 30 per week)	Fruit (2-3 Servings per day)	Processed Foods (Avoid / Minimize)

Daily Journal / Reflection Page

Date: _____

Today I am grateful for:

- _____
- _____
- _____

Important Tasks for Today:

_____
_____
_____

One thing that made me feel proud / happy:

_____

One thing that made me stressed / challenged:

_____

Daily Reflection:

_____
_____
_____
_____
_____
_____
_____

DAILY FOOD JOURNAL

Current Weight:

Breakfast: _____ am

Lunch: _____ pm

Dinner _____ pm

Snacks

Vegetables (Target 30 per week)	Fruit (2-3 Servings per day)	Processed Foods (Avoid / Minimize)

Daily Journal / Reflection Page

Date: _____

Today I am grateful for:

- _____
- _____
- _____

Important Tasks for Today:

_____
_____
_____

One thing that made me feel proud / happy:

_____

One thing that made me stressed / challenged:

_____

Daily Reflection:

_____
_____
_____
_____
_____
_____
_____
_____

DAILY FOOD JOURNAL

Current Weight: _____

Breakfast: _____ am
Lunch: _____ pm
Dinner _____ pm
Snacks

Vegetables (Target 30 per week)	Fruit (2-3 Servings per day)	Processed Foods (Avoid / Minimize)

Deep Reflection Prompts

Use these prompts inspired by Jerry Colonna when you feel the need for deeper introspection:

- How have I been complicit in creating the condition I say I do not want?

- What am I not saying that needs to be said?

- What is being said that I am not hearing?

- Right now, I am feeling…

- In what ways do I deplete myself and run myself into the ground?

- Where am I running from and where am I running to?

Weekly Review Prompts

- What progress have I made this week on my habits?

- Where did I feel most energized?

- What challenges did I face, and how did I respond?

- What could I improve for next week?

- Which habit or mindset helped me most?

Top 3 Goals for the Coming Week:

1.
2.
3.

"Tell me who you spend your time with, and I will tell you who you are."

– *Goethe*

Weekly Habit Tracker

Track your habits using the **SHAVE GAMERS** framework. Use this weekly template to keep yourself accountable:

Habits:	Monday	Tuesday	Wednesday	Thursday	Friday	Saturday	Sunday
Sleep							
Hydration							
Affirmations							
Visualizations							
Exercise							
Gratitude							
Audible / Learning							
Meditation							
Eat Healthy							
Relationships							
Scribing							

WEEKLY FITNESS TRACKER

Monday	Daily Steps:	Duration:
Workout		

Tuesday	Daily Steps:	Duration:
Workout		

Wednesday	Daily Steps:	Duration:
Workout		

Thursday	Daily Steps:	Duration:
Workout		

Friday	Daily Steps:	Duration:
Workout		

Saturday	Daily Steps:	Duration:
Workout		

Sunday	Daily Steps:	Duration:
Workout		

Daily Journal / Reflection Page

Date: _____

Today I am grateful for:

- _____
- _____
- _____

Important Tasks for Today:

_____
_____
_____

One thing that made me feel proud / happy:

_____

One thing that made me stressed / challenged:

_____

Daily Reflection:

_____
_____
_____
_____
_____
_____
_____

DAILY FOOD JOURNAL

Current Weight:

Breakfast: _____ am
Lunch: _____ pm
Dinner _____ pm
Snacks

Vegetables (Target 30 per week)	Fruit (2-3 Servings per day)	Processed Foods (Avoid / Minimize)

Daily Journal / Reflection Page

Date: _____

Today I am grateful for:

- _____
- _____
- _____

Important Tasks for Today:

_____

_____

_____

_____

One thing that made me feel proud / happy:

_____

One thing that made me stressed / challenged:

_____

Daily Reflection:

_____

_____

_____

_____

_____

_____

_____

DAILY FOOD JOURNAL

<u>Current Weight:</u>

Breakfast: _____ am

Lunch: _____ pm

Dinner _____ pm

Snacks

Vegetables (Target 30 per week)	Fruit (2-3 Servings per day)	Processed Foods (Avoid / Minimize)

Daily Journal / Reflection Page

Date: _____

Today I am grateful for:

- _____
- _____
- _____

Important Tasks for Today:

_____
_____
_____

One thing that made me feel proud / happy:

_____

One thing that made me stressed / challenged:

_____

Daily Reflection:

_____
_____
_____
_____
_____
_____
_____

DAILY FOOD JOURNAL

Current Weight:

Breakfast: _____ am

Lunch: _____ pm

Dinner _____ pm

Snacks

Vegetables (Target 30 per week)	Fruit (2-3 Servings per day)	Processed Foods (Avoid / Minimize)

Daily Journal / Reflection Page

Date: _____

Today I am grateful for:

- _____
- _____
- _____

Important Tasks for Today:

_____
_____
_____

One thing that made me feel proud / happy:

_____

One thing that made me stressed / challenged:

_____

Daily Reflection:

_____
_____
_____
_____
_____
_____
_____
_____

DAILY FOOD JOURNAL

Current Weight:

Breakfast: _____ am

Lunch: _____ pm

Dinner _____ pm

Snacks

Vegetables (Target 30 per week)	Fruit (2-3 Servings per day)	Processed Foods (Avoid / Minimize)

Daily Journal / Reflection Page

Date: _____

Today I am grateful for:

- _____
- _____
- _____

Important Tasks for Today:

_____
_____
_____

One thing that made me feel proud / happy:

_____

One thing that made me stressed / challenged:

_____

Daily Reflection:

_____
_____
_____
_____
_____
_____
_____

DAILY FOOD JOURNAL

Current Weight:

Breakfast: _____ am

Lunch: _____ pm

Dinner _____ pm

Snacks

Vegetables (Target 30 per week)	Fruit (2-3 Servings per day)	Processed Foods (Avoid / Minimize)

Daily Journal / Reflection Page

Date: _____

Today I am grateful for:

- _____
- _____
- _____

Important Tasks for Today:

_____
_____
_____

One thing that made me feel proud / happy:

_____

One thing that made me stressed / challenged:

_____

Daily Reflection:

_____
_____
_____
_____
_____
_____
_____
_____

DAILY FOOD JOURNAL

Current Weight:

Breakfast: _____ am

Lunch: _____ pm

Dinner _____ pm

Snacks

Vegetables (Target 30 per week)	Fruit (2-3 Servings per day)	Processed Foods (Avoid / Minimize)

Daily Journal / Reflection Page

Date: _____

Today I am grateful for:

- _____
- _____
- _____

Important Tasks for Today:

_____
_____
_____

One thing that made me feel proud / happy:

_____

One thing that made me stressed / challenged:

_____

Daily Reflection:

_____
_____
_____
_____
_____
_____
_____

DAILY FOOD JOURNAL

Current Weight:

Breakfast: _____ am

Lunch: _____ pm

Dinner _____ pm

Snacks

Vegetables (Target 30 per week)	Fruit (2-3 Servings per day)	Processed Foods (Avoid / Minimize)

Deep Reflection Prompts

Use these prompts inspired by Jerry Colonna when you feel the need for deeper introspection:

- How have I been complicit in creating the condition I say I do not want?

  _____
  _____

- What am I not saying that needs to be said?

  _____
  _____

- What is being said that I am not hearing?

  _____
  _____

- Right now, I am feeling…

  _____
  _____

- In what ways do I deplete myself and run myself into the ground?

  _____
  _____

- Where am I running from and where am I running to?

  _____
  _____

Weekly Review Prompts

- What progress have I made this week on my habits?

  _____
  _____

- Where did I feel most energized?

  _____
  _____

- What challenges did I face, and how did I respond?

  _____
  _____

- What could I improve for next week?

  _____
  _____

- Which habit or mindset helped me most?

  _____
  _____

Top 3 Goals for the Coming Week:

1. _____
2. _____
3. _____

"Find something that feels like play to you but looks like work to others."

– Naval Ravikant

Weekly Habit Tracker

Track your habits using the SHAVE GAMERS framework. Use this weekly template to keep yourself accountable:

Habits:	Monday	Tuesday	Wednesday	Thursday	Friday	Saturday	Sunday
Sleep							
Hydration							
Affirmations							
Visualizations							
Exercise							
Gratitude							
Audible / Learning							
Meditation							
Eat Healthy							
Relationships							
Scribing							

WEEKLY FITNESS TRACKER

Monday	Daily Steps:	Duration:
Workout		

Tuesday	Daily Steps:	Duration:
Workout		

Wednesday	Daily Steps:	Duration:
Workout		

Thursday	Daily Steps:	Duration:
Workout		

Friday	Daily Steps:	Duration:
Workout		

Saturday	Daily Steps:	Duration:
Workout		

Sunday	Daily Steps:	Duration:
Workout		

Daily Journal / Reflection Page

Date: _____

Today I am grateful for:

- _____
- _____
- _____

Important Tasks for Today:

_____
_____
_____

One thing that made me feel proud / happy:

_____

One thing that made me stressed / challenged:

_____

Daily Reflection:

_____
_____
_____
_____
_____
_____
_____

DAILY FOOD JOURNAL

Current Weight: _____

Breakfast: _____ am

Lunch: _____ pm

Dinner _____ pm

Snacks

Vegetables (Target 30 per week)	Fruit (2-3 Servings per day)	Processed Foods (Avoid / Minimize)

Daily Journal / Reflection Page

Date: _____

Today I am grateful for:

- _____
- _____
- _____

Important Tasks for Today:

_____
_____
_____
_____

One thing that made me feel proud / happy:

_____

One thing that made me stressed / challenged:

_____

Daily Reflection:

_____
_____
_____
_____
_____
_____
_____
_____

DAILY FOOD JOURNAL

Current Weight:

Breakfast: _____ am

Lunch: _____ pm

Dinner _____ pm

Snacks

Vegetables (Target 30 per week)	Fruit (2-3 Servings per day)	Processed Foods (Avoid / Minimize)

Daily Journal / Reflection Page

Date: _____

Today I am grateful for:

- _____
- _____
- _____

Important Tasks for Today:

_____
_____
_____

One thing that made me feel proud / happy:

_____

One thing that made me stressed / challenged:

_____

Daily Reflection:

_____
_____
_____
_____
_____
_____
_____
_____

DAILY FOOD JOURNAL

Current Weight:

Breakfast: _____ am

Lunch: _____ pm

Dinner _____ pm

Snacks

Vegetables (Target 30 per week)	Fruit (2-3 Servings per day)	Processed Foods (Avoid / Minimize)

Daily Journal / Reflection Page

Date: _____

Today I am grateful for:

- _____
- _____
- _____

Important Tasks for Today:

_____
_____
_____

One thing that made me feel proud / happy:

_____

One thing that made me stressed / challenged:

_____

Daily Reflection:

_____
_____
_____
_____
_____
_____
_____

DAILY FOOD JOURNAL

Current Weight:

Breakfast: _____ am

Lunch: _____ pm

Dinner _____ pm

Snacks

Vegetables (Target 30 per week)	Fruit (2-3 Servings per day)	Processed Foods (Avoid / Minimize)

Daily Journal / Reflection Page

Date: _____

Today I am grateful for:

- _____
- _____
- _____

Important Tasks for Today:

_____
_____
_____

One thing that made me feel proud / happy:

_____

One thing that made me stressed / challenged:

_____

Daily Reflection:

_____
_____
_____
_____
_____
_____
_____
_____

DAILY FOOD JOURNAL

Current Weight: _____

Breakfast: _____ am

Lunch: _____ pm

Dinner _____ pm

Snacks

Vegetables (Target 30 per week)	Fruit (2-3 Servings per day)	Processed Foods (Avoid / Minimize)

Daily Journal / Reflection Page

Date: _____

Today I am grateful for:

- _____
- _____
- _____

Important Tasks for Today:

_____
_____
_____

One thing that made me feel proud / happy:

_____

One thing that made me stressed / challenged:

_____

Daily Reflection:

_____
_____
_____
_____
_____
_____
_____
_____

DAILY FOOD JOURNAL

Current Weight:

Breakfast: _____am

Lunch: _____pm

Dinner _____pm

Snacks

Vegetables (Target 30 per week)	Fruit (2-3 Servings per day)	Processed Foods (Avoid / Minimize)

Daily Journal / Reflection Page

Date: _____

Today I am grateful for:

- _____
- _____
- _____

Important Tasks for Today:

_____
_____
_____

One thing that made me feel proud / happy:

_____

One thing that made me stressed / challenged:

_____

Daily Reflection:

_____
_____
_____
_____
_____
_____
_____
_____

DAILY FOOD JOURNAL

Current Weight:

Breakfast: _____ am

Lunch: _____ pm

Dinner _____ pm

Snacks

Vegetables (Target 30 per week)	Fruit (2-3 Servings per day)	Processed Foods (Avoid / Minimize)

Deep Reflection Prompts

Use these prompts inspired by Jerry Colonna when you feel the need for deeper introspection:

- How have I been complicit in creating the condition I say I do not want?

  _____
  _____

- What am I not saying that needs to be said?

  _____
  _____

- What is being said that I am not hearing?

  _____
  _____

- Right now, I am feeling…

  _____
  _____

- In what ways do I deplete myself and run myself into the ground?

  _____
  _____

- Where am I running from and where am I running to?

  _____
  _____

Weekly Review Prompts

- What progress have I made this week on my habits?

  _____
  _____

- Where did I feel most energized?

  _____
  _____

- What challenges did I face, and how did I respond?

  _____
  _____

- What could I improve for next week?

  _____
  _____

- Which habit or mindset helped me most?

  _____
  _____

Top 3 Goals for the Coming Week:

1. _____
2. _____
3. _____

"Life punishes the vague wish and rewards the specific ask."

– Tim Ferriss

Weekly Habit Tracker

Track your habits using the **SHAVE GAMERS** framework. Use this weekly template to keep yourself accountable:

Habits:	Monday	Tuesday	Wednesday	Thursday	Friday	Saturday	Sunday
Sleep							
Hydration							
Affirmations							
Visualizations							
Exercise							
Gratitude							
Audible / Learning							
Meditation							
Eat Healthy							
Relationships							
Scribing							

WEEKLY FITNESS TRACKER

Monday	Daily Steps:	Duration:
Workout		

Tuesday	Daily Steps:	Duration:
Workout		

Wednesday	Daily Steps:	Duration:
Workout		

Thursday	Daily Steps:	Duration:
Workout		

Friday	Daily Steps:	Duration:
Workout		

Saturday	Daily Steps:	Duration:
Workout		

Sunday	Daily Steps:	Duration:
Workout		

Daily Journal / Reflection Page

Date: _____

Today I am grateful for:

- _____
- _____
- _____

Important Tasks for Today:

_____
_____
_____

One thing that made me feel proud / happy:

_____

One thing that made me stressed / challenged:

_____

Daily Reflection:

_____
_____
_____
_____
_____
_____
_____
_____

DAILY FOOD JOURNAL

Current Weight:

Breakfast: _____ am

Lunch: _____ pm

Dinner _____ pm

Snacks

Vegetables (Target 30 per week)	Fruit (2-3 Servings per day)	Processed Foods (Avoid / Minimize)

Daily Journal / Reflection Page

Date: _____

Today I am grateful for:

- _____
- _____
- _____

Important Tasks for Today:

_____
_____
_____

One thing that made me feel proud / happy:

_____

One thing that made me stressed / challenged:

_____

Daily Reflection:

_____
_____
_____
_____
_____
_____
_____
_____

DAILY FOOD JOURNAL

Current Weight:

Breakfast: _____ am

Lunch: _____ pm

Dinner _____ pm

Snacks

Vegetables (Target 30 per week)	Fruit (2-3 Servings per day)	Processed Foods (Avoid / Minimize)

Daily Journal / Reflection Page

Date: _____

Today I am grateful for:

- _____
- _____
- _____

Important Tasks for Today:

_____
_____
_____

One thing that made me feel proud / happy:

_____

One thing that made me stressed / challenged:

_____

Daily Reflection:

_____
_____
_____
_____
_____
_____
_____

DAILY FOOD JOURNAL

Current Weight:

Breakfast: _____am

Lunch: _____pm

Dinner _____pm

Snacks

Vegetables (Target 30 per week)	Fruit (2-3 Servings per day)	Processed Foods (Avoid / Minimize)

Daily Journal / Reflection Page

Date: _____

Today I am grateful for:

- _____
- _____
- _____

Important Tasks for Today:

_____
_____
_____

One thing that made me feel proud / happy:

_____

One thing that made me stressed / challenged:

_____

Daily Reflection:

_____
_____
_____
_____
_____
_____
_____

DAILY FOOD JOURNAL

Current Weight:

Breakfast: _____ am

Lunch: _____ pm

Dinner _____ pm

Snacks

Vegetables (Target 30 per week)	Fruit (2-3 Servings per day)	Processed Foods (Avoid / Minimize)

Daily Journal / Reflection Page

Date: _____

Today I am grateful for:

- _____
- _____
- _____

Important Tasks for Today:

_____
_____
_____

One thing that made me feel proud / happy:

_____

One thing that made me stressed / challenged:

_____

Daily Reflection:

_____
_____
_____
_____
_____
_____
_____

DAILY FOOD JOURNAL

Current Weight: _____

Breakfast: _____ am

Lunch: _____ pm

Dinner _____ pm

Snacks

Vegetables (Target 30 per week)	Fruit (2-3 Servings per day)	Processed Foods (Avoid / Minimize)

Daily Journal / Reflection Page

Date: _____

Today I am grateful for:

- _____
- _____
- _____

Important Tasks for Today:

_____
_____
_____
_____

One thing that made me feel proud / happy:

_____

One thing that made me stressed / challenged:

_____

Daily Reflection:

_____
_____
_____
_____
_____
_____
_____
_____

DAILY FOOD JOURNAL

Current Weight:

Breakfast: _____ am

Lunch: _____ pm

Dinner _____ pm

Snacks

Vegetables (Target 30 per week)	Fruit (2-3 Servings per day)	Processed Foods (Avoid / Minimize)

Daily Journal / Reflection Page

Date: _____

Today I am grateful for:

- _____
- _____
- _____

Important Tasks for Today:

_____
_____
_____

One thing that made me feel proud / happy:

_____

One thing that made me stressed / challenged:

_____

Daily Reflection:

_____
_____
_____
_____
_____
_____
_____
_____

DAILY FOOD JOURNAL

Current Weight:

Breakfast: _____am

Lunch: _____pm

Dinner _____pm

Snacks

Vegetables (Target 30 per week)	Fruit (2-3 Servings per day)	Processed Foods (Avoid / Minimize)

Deep Reflection Prompts

Use these prompts inspired by Jerry Colonna when you feel the need for deeper introspection:

- How have I been complicit in creating the condition I say I do not want?

  _____
  _____

- What am I not saying that needs to be said?

  _____
  _____

- What is being said that I am not hearing?

  _____
  _____

- Right now, I am feeling…

  _____
  _____

- In what ways do I deplete myself and run myself into the ground?

  _____
  _____

- Where am I running from and where am I running to?

  _____
  _____

Weekly Review Prompts

- What progress have I made this week on my habits?
  _____
  _____

- Where did I feel most energized?
  _____
  _____

- What challenges did I face, and how did I respond?
  _____
  _____

- What could I improve for next week?
  _____
  _____

- Which habit or mindset helped me most?
  _____
  _____

Top 3 Goals for the Coming Week:

1. _____
2. _____
3. _____

"The modern mind is overstimulated, and the modern body is understimulated, and overfed. Meditation, exercise, and fasting restore an ancient balance."

– *Naval Ravikant*

Weekly Habit Tracker

Track your habits using the **SHAVE GAMERS** framework. Use this weekly template to keep yourself accountable:

Habits:	Monday	Tuesday	Wednesday	Thursday	Friday	Saturday	Sunday
Sleep							
Hydration							
Affirmations							
Visualizations							
Exercise							
Gratitude							
Audible / Learning							
Meditation							
Eat Healthy							
Relationships							
Scribing							

WEEKLY FITNESS TRACKER

Monday	Daily Steps:	Duration:
Workout		

Tuesday	Daily Steps:	Duration:
Workout		

Wednesday	Daily Steps:	Duration:
Workout		

Thursday	Daily Steps:	Duration:
Workout		

Friday	Daily Steps:	Duration:
Workout		

Saturday	Daily Steps:	Duration:
Workout		

Sunday	Daily Steps:	Duration:
Workout		

Daily Journal / Reflection Page

Date: _____

Today I am grateful for:

- _____
- _____
- _____

Important Tasks for Today:

_____
_____
_____

One thing that made me feel proud / happy:

_____

One thing that made me stressed / challenged:

_____

Daily Reflection:

_____
_____
_____
_____
_____
_____
_____
_____

DAILY FOOD JOURNAL

Current Weight: _____

Breakfast: _____ am

Lunch: _____ pm

Dinner _____ pm

Snacks

Vegetables (Target 30 per week)	Fruit (2-3 Servings per day)	Processed Foods (Avoid / Minimize)

Daily Journal / Reflection Page

Date: _____

Today I am grateful for:

- _____
- _____
- _____

Important Tasks for Today:

_____
_____
_____

One thing that made me feel proud / happy:

_____

One thing that made me stressed / challenged:

_____

Daily Reflection:

_____
_____
_____
_____
_____
_____
_____
_____

DAILY FOOD JOURNAL

Current Weight: _____

Breakfast: _____ am
Lunch: _____ pm
Dinner _____ pm
Snacks

Vegetables (Target 30 per week)	Fruit (2-3 Servings per day)	Processed Foods (Avoid / Minimize)

Daily Journal / Reflection Page

Date: _____

Today I am grateful for:

- _____
- _____
- _____

Important Tasks for Today:

_____
_____
_____
_____

One thing that made me feel proud / happy:

_____

One thing that made me stressed / challenged:

_____

Daily Reflection:

_____
_____
_____
_____
_____
_____
_____
_____

DAILY FOOD JOURNAL

Current Weight:

Breakfast: _____ am

Lunch: _____ pm

Dinner _____ pm

Snacks

Vegetables (Target 30 per week)	Fruit (2-3 Servings per day)	Processed Foods (Avoid / Minimize)

Daily Journal / Reflection Page

Date: _____

Today I am grateful for:

- _____
- _____
- _____

Important Tasks for Today:

_____
_____
_____

One thing that made me feel proud / happy:

_____

One thing that made me stressed / challenged:

_____

Daily Reflection:

_____
_____
_____
_____
_____
_____
_____
_____

DAILY FOOD JOURNAL

Current Weight: _____

Breakfast: _____am

Lunch: _____pm

Dinner _____pm

Snacks

Vegetables (Target 30 per week)	Fruit (2-3 Servings per day)	Processed Foods (Avoid / Minimize)

Daily Journal / Reflection Page

Date: _____

Today I am grateful for:

- _____
- _____
- _____

Important Tasks for Today:

_____
_____
_____

One thing that made me feel proud / happy:

_____

One thing that made me stressed / challenged:

_____

Daily Reflection:

_____
_____
_____
_____
_____
_____
_____
_____

DAILY FOOD JOURNAL

Current Weight:

Breakfast: _____ am

Lunch: _____ pm

Dinner _____ pm

Snacks

Vegetables (Target 30 per week)	Fruit (2-3 Servings per day)	Processed Foods (Avoid / Minimize)

Daily Journal / Reflection Page

Date: _____

Today I am grateful for:

- _____
- _____
- _____

Important Tasks for Today:

_____
_____
_____

One thing that made me feel proud / happy:

_____

One thing that made me stressed / challenged:

_____

Daily Reflection:

_____
_____
_____
_____
_____
_____
_____
_____

DAILY FOOD JOURNAL

Current Weight: _____

Breakfast: _____am

Lunch: _____pm

Dinner _____pm

Snacks

Vegetables (Target 30 per week)	Fruit (2-3 Servings per day)	Processed Foods (Avoid / Minimize)

Daily Journal / Reflection Page

Date: _____

Today I am grateful for:

- _____
- _____
- _____

Important Tasks for Today:

_____
_____
_____

One thing that made me feel proud / happy:

_____

One thing that made me stressed / challenged:

_____

Daily Reflection:

_____
_____
_____
_____
_____
_____
_____
_____

DAILY FOOD JOURNAL

Current Weight:

Breakfast: _____ am

Lunch: _____ pm

Dinner _____ pm

Snacks

Vegetables (Target 30 per week)	Fruit (2-3 Servings per day)	Processed Foods (Avoid / Minimize)

Deep Reflection Prompts

Use these prompts inspired by Jerry Colonna when you feel the need for deeper introspection:

- How have I been complicit in creating the condition I say I do not want?

  _____
  _____

- What am I not saying that needs to be said?

  _____
  _____

- What is being said that I am not hearing?

  _____
  _____

- Right now, I am feeling…

  _____
  _____

- In what ways do I deplete myself and run myself into the ground?

  _____
  _____

- Where am I running from and where am I running to?

  _____
  _____

Weekly Review Prompts

- What progress have I made this week on my habits?
  _____
  _____

- Where did I feel most energized?
  _____
  _____

- What challenges did I face, and how did I respond?
  _____
  _____

- What could I improve for next week?
  _____
  _____

- Which habit or mindset helped me most?
  _____
  _____

Top 3 Goals for the Coming Week:

1. _____
2. _____
3. _____

"You won't act differently until you think of yourself differently."

– Derek Sivers

Weekly Habit Tracker

Track your habits using the SHAVE GAMERS framework. Use this weekly template to keep yourself accountable:

Habits:	Monday	Tuesday	Wednesday	Thursday	Friday	Saturday	Sunday
Sleep							
Hydration							
Affirmations							
Visualizations							
Exercise							
Gratitude							
Audible / Learning							
Meditation							
Eat Healthy							
Relationships							
Scribing							

WEEKLY FITNESS TRACKER

Monday	Daily Steps:	Duration:
Workout		

Tuesday	Daily Steps:	Duration:
Workout		

Wednesday	Daily Steps:	Duration:
Workout		

Thursday	Daily Steps:	Duration:
Workout		

Friday	Daily Steps:	Duration:
Workout		

Saturday	Daily Steps:	Duration:
Workout		

Sunday	Daily Steps:	Duration:
Workout		

Daily Journal / Reflection Page

Date: _____

Today I am grateful for:

- _____
- _____
- _____

Important Tasks for Today:

_____
_____
_____

One thing that made me feel proud / happy:

_____

One thing that made me stressed / challenged:

_____

Daily Reflection:

_____
_____
_____
_____
_____
_____
_____

DAILY FOOD JOURNAL

Current Weight:

Breakfast: _____am

Lunch: _____pm

Dinner _____pm

Snacks

Vegetables (Target 30 per week)	Fruit (2-3 Servings per day)	Processed Foods (Avoid / Minimize)

Daily Journal / Reflection Page

Date: _____

Today I am grateful for:

- _____
- _____
- _____

Important Tasks for Today:

_____
_____
_____

One thing that made me feel proud / happy:

_____

One thing that made me stressed / challenged:

_____

Daily Reflection:

_____
_____
_____
_____
_____
_____
_____
_____

DAILY FOOD JOURNAL

Current Weight:

Breakfast: _____ am

Lunch: _____ pm

Dinner _____ pm

Snacks

Vegetables (Target 30 per week)	Fruit (2-3 Servings per day)	Processed Foods (Avoid / Minimize)

Daily Journal / Reflection Page

Date: _____

Today I am grateful for:

- _____
- _____
- _____

Important Tasks for Today:

_____
_____
_____

One thing that made me feel proud / happy:

_____

One thing that made me stressed / challenged:

_____

Daily Reflection:

_____
_____
_____
_____
_____
_____
_____

DAILY FOOD JOURNAL

Current Weight: _____

Breakfast: _____am

Lunch: _____pm

Dinner _____pm

Snacks

Vegetables (Target 30 per week)	Fruit (2-3 Servings per day)	Processed Foods (Avoid / Minimize)

Daily Journal / Reflection Page

Date: _____

Today I am grateful for:

- _____
- _____
- _____

Important Tasks for Today:

_____
_____
_____
_____

One thing that made me feel proud / happy:

_____

One thing that made me stressed / challenged:

_____

Daily Reflection:

_____
_____
_____
_____
_____
_____
_____

DAILY FOOD JOURNAL

Current Weight:

Breakfast: _____am

Lunch: _____pm

Dinner _____pm

Snacks

Vegetables (Target 30 per week)	Fruit (2-3 Servings per day)	Processed Foods (Avoid / Minimize)

Daily Journal / Reflection Page

Date: _____

Today I am grateful for:

- _____
- _____
- _____

Important Tasks for Today:

_____
_____
_____

One thing that made me feel proud / happy:

_____

One thing that made me stressed / challenged:

_____

Daily Reflection:

_____
_____
_____
_____
_____
_____
_____

DAILY FOOD JOURNAL

Current Weight:

Breakfast: _____ am

Lunch: _____ pm

Dinner _____ pm

Snacks

Vegetables (Target 30 per week)	Fruit (2-3 Servings per day)	Processed Foods (Avoid / Minimize)

Daily Journal / Reflection Page

Date: _____

Today I am grateful for:

- _____
- _____
- _____

Important Tasks for Today:

_____
_____
_____

One thing that made me feel proud / happy:

_____

One thing that made me stressed / challenged:

_____

Daily Reflection:

_____
_____
_____
_____
_____
_____
_____
_____

DAILY FOOD JOURNAL

Current Weight:

Breakfast: _____ am

Lunch: _____ pm

Dinner _____ pm

Snacks

Vegetables (Target 30 per week)	Fruit (2-3 Servings per day)	Processed Foods (Avoid / Minimize)

Daily Journal / Reflection Page

Date: _____

Today I am grateful for:

- _____
- _____
- _____

Important Tasks for Today:

_____
_____
_____

One thing that made me feel proud / happy:

_____

One thing that made me stressed / challenged:

_____

Daily Reflection:

_____
_____
_____
_____
_____
_____
_____

DAILY FOOD JOURNAL

Current Weight:

Breakfast: _____ am

Lunch: _____ pm

Dinner _____ pm

Snacks

Vegetables (Target 30 per week)	Fruit (2-3 Servings per day)	Processed Foods (Avoid / Minimize)

Deep Reflection Prompts

Use these prompts inspired by Jerry Colonna when you feel the need for deeper introspection:

- How have I been complicit in creating the condition I say I do not want?

- What am I not saying that needs to be said?

- What is being said that I am not hearing?

- Right now, I am feeling…

- In what ways do I deplete myself and run myself into the ground?

- Where am I running from and where am I running to?

Weekly Review Prompts

- What progress have I made this week on my habits?
  _____
  _____

- Where did I feel most energized?
  _____
  _____

- What challenges did I face, and how did I respond?
  _____
  _____

- What could I improve for next week?
  _____
  _____

- Which habit or mindset helped me most?
  _____
  _____

Top 3 Goals for the Coming Week:

1. _____
2. _____
3. _____

"You don't succeed because you have no weaknesses, you succeed because you find your unique strengths and focus on developing habits around them."

— Tim Ferriss

Weekly Habit Tracker

Track your habits using the **SHAVE GAMERS** framework. Use this weekly template to keep yourself accountable:

Habits:	Monday	Tuesday	Wednesday	Thursday	Friday	Saturday	Sunday
Sleep							
Hydration							
Affirmations							
Visualizations							
Exercise							
Gratitude							
Audible / Learning							
Meditation							
Eat Healthy							
Relationships							
Scribing							

WEEKLY FITNESS TRACKER

Monday	Daily Steps:	Duration:
Workout		

Tuesday	Daily Steps:	Duration:
Workout		

Wednesday	Daily Steps:	Duration:
Workout		

Thursday	Daily Steps:	Duration:
Workout		

Friday	Daily Steps:	Duration:
Workout		

Saturday	Daily Steps:	Duration:
Workout		

Sunday	Daily Steps:	Duration:
Workout		

Daily Journal / Reflection Page

Date: _____

Today I am grateful for:

- _____
- _____
- _____

Important Tasks for Today:

_____
_____
_____

One thing that made me feel proud / happy:

_____

One thing that made me stressed / challenged:

_____

Daily Reflection:

_____
_____
_____
_____
_____
_____
_____

DAILY FOOD JOURNAL

Current Weight:

Breakfast: _____ am

Lunch: _____ pm

Dinner _____ pm

Snacks

Vegetables (Target 30 per week)	Fruit (2-3 Servings per day)	Processed Foods (Avoid / Minimize)

Daily Journal / Reflection Page

Date: _____

Today I am grateful for:

- _____
- _____
- _____

Important Tasks for Today:

_____
_____
_____

One thing that made me feel proud / happy:

_____

One thing that made me stressed / challenged:

_____

Daily Reflection:

_____
_____
_____
_____
_____
_____
_____

DAILY FOOD JOURNAL

Current Weight:

Breakfast: _____ am

Lunch: _____ pm

Dinner _____ pm

Snacks

Vegetables (Target 30 per week)	Fruit (2-3 Servings per day)	Processed Foods (Avoid / Minimize)

Daily Journal / Reflection Page

Date: _____

Today I am grateful for:

- _____
- _____
- _____

Important Tasks for Today:

_____
_____
_____

One thing that made me feel proud / happy:

_____

One thing that made me stressed / challenged:

_____

Daily Reflection:

_____
_____
_____
_____
_____
_____
_____
_____

DAILY FOOD JOURNAL

Current Weight:

Breakfast: _____ am

Lunch: _____ pm

Dinner _____ pm

Snacks

Vegetables (Target 30 per week)	Fruit (2-3 Servings per day)	Processed Foods (Avoid / Minimize)

Daily Journal / Reflection Page

Date: _____

Today I am grateful for:

- _____
- _____
- _____

Important Tasks for Today:

_____
_____
_____

One thing that made me feel proud / happy:

_____

One thing that made me stressed / challenged:

_____

Daily Reflection:

_____
_____
_____
_____
_____
_____
_____

DAILY FOOD JOURNAL

Current Weight: _____

Breakfast: _____am

Lunch: _____pm

Dinner _____pm

Snacks

Vegetables (Target 30 per week)	Fruit (2-3 Servings per day)	Processed Foods (Avoid / Minimize)

Daily Journal / Reflection Page

Date: _____

Today I am grateful for:

- _____
- _____
- _____

Important Tasks for Today:

_____
_____
_____

One thing that made me feel proud / happy:

_____

One thing that made me stressed / challenged:

_____

Daily Reflection:

_____
_____
_____
_____
_____
_____
_____
_____

DAILY FOOD JOURNAL

Current Weight:

Breakfast: _____ am

Lunch: _____ pm

Dinner _____ pm

Snacks

Vegetables (Target 30 per week)	Fruit (2-3 Servings per day)	Processed Foods (Avoid / Minimize)

Daily Journal / Reflection Page

Date: _____

Today I am grateful for:

- _____
- _____
- _____

Important Tasks for Today:

_____
_____
_____

One thing that made me feel proud / happy:

_____

One thing that made me stressed / challenged:

_____

Daily Reflection:

_____
_____
_____
_____
_____
_____
_____

DAILY FOOD JOURNAL

Current Weight:

Breakfast: _____am
Lunch: _____pm
Dinner _____pm
Snacks

Vegetables (Target 30 per week)	Fruit (2-3 Servings per day)	Processed Foods (Avoid / Minimize)

Daily Journal / Reflection Page

Date: _____

Today I am grateful for:

- _____
- _____
- _____

Important Tasks for Today:

_____
_____
_____

One thing that made me feel proud / happy:

_____

One thing that made me stressed / challenged:

_____

Daily Reflection:

_____
_____
_____
_____
_____
_____
_____
_____

DAILY FOOD JOURNAL

Current Weight:

Breakfast: _____ am

Lunch: _____ pm

Dinner _____ pm

Snacks

Vegetables (Target 30 per week)	Fruit (2-3 Servings per day)	Processed Foods (Avoid / Minimize)

Deep Reflection Prompts

Use these prompts inspired by Jerry Colonna when you feel the need for deeper introspection:

- How have I been complicit in creating the condition I say I do not want?

  _____
  _____

- What am I not saying that needs to be said?

  _____
  _____

- What is being said that I am not hearing?

  _____
  _____

- Right now, I am feeling…

  _____
  _____

- In what ways do I deplete myself and run myself into the ground?

  _____
  _____

- Where am I running from and where am I running to?

  _____
  _____

Weekly Review Prompts

- What progress have I made this week on my habits?
  _____
  _____

- Where did I feel most energized?
  _____
  _____

- What challenges did I face, and how did I respond?
  _____
  _____

- What could I improve for next week?
  _____
  _____

- Which habit or mindset helped me most?
  _____
  _____

Top 3 Goals for the Coming Week:

1. _____
2. _____
3. _____

"If a man looks at the world at fifty the same way he did when he was twenty and hasn't changed, he's wasted thirty years of his life."

— Mohammad Ali

Weekly Habit Tracker

Track your habits using the SHAVE GAMERS framework. Use this weekly template to keep yourself accountable:

Habits:	Monday	Tuesday	Wednesday	Thursday	Friday	Saturday	Sunday
Sleep							
Hydration							
Affirmations							
Visualizations							
Exercise							
Gratitude							
Audible / Learning							
Meditation							
Eat Healthy							
Relationships							
Scribing							

WEEKLY FITNESS TRACKER

Monday	Daily Steps:	Duration:
Workout		

Tuesday	Daily Steps:	Duration:
Workout		

Wednesday	Daily Steps:	Duration:
Workout		

Thursday	Daily Steps:	Duration:
Workout		

Friday	Daily Steps:	Duration:
Workout		

Saturday	Daily Steps:	Duration:
Workout		

Sunday	Daily Steps:	Duration:
Workout		

Daily Journal / Reflection Page

Date: _____

Today I am grateful for:

- _____
- _____
- _____

Important Tasks for Today:

_____
_____
_____

One thing that made me feel proud / happy:

_____

One thing that made me stressed / challenged:

_____

Daily Reflection:

_____
_____
_____
_____
_____
_____
_____

DAILY FOOD JOURNAL

Current Weight: _____

Breakfast: _____ am

Lunch: _____ pm

Dinner _____ pm

Snacks

Vegetables (Target 30 per week)	Fruit (2-3 Servings per day)	Processed Foods (Avoid / Minimize)

Daily Journal / Reflection Page

Date: _____

Today I am grateful for:

- _____
- _____
- _____

Important Tasks for Today:

_____
_____
_____

One thing that made me feel proud / happy:

_____

One thing that made me stressed / challenged:

_____

Daily Reflection:

_____
_____
_____
_____
_____
_____
_____
_____

DAILY FOOD JOURNAL

Current Weight:

Breakfast: _____am

Lunch: _____pm

Dinner _____pm

Snacks

Vegetables (Target 30 per week)	Fruit (2-3 Servings per day)	Processed Foods (Avoid / Minimize)

Daily Journal / Reflection Page

Date: _____

Today I am grateful for:

- _____
- _____
- _____

Important Tasks for Today:

_____
_____
_____

One thing that made me feel proud / happy:

_____

One thing that made me stressed / challenged:

_____

Daily Reflection:

_____
_____
_____
_____
_____
_____
_____
_____

DAILY FOOD JOURNAL

Current Weight: _____

Breakfast: _____am

Lunch: _____pm

Dinner _____pm

Snacks

Vegetables (Target 30 per week)	Fruit (2-3 Servings per day)	Processed Foods (Avoid / Minimize)

Daily Journal / Reflection Page

Date: _____

Today I am grateful for:

- _____
- _____
- _____

Important Tasks for Today:

_____
_____
_____

One thing that made me feel proud / happy:

_____

One thing that made me stressed / challenged:

_____

Daily Reflection:

_____
_____
_____
_____
_____
_____
_____
_____

DAILY FOOD JOURNAL

Current Weight:

Breakfast: _____am

Lunch: _____pm

Dinner _____pm

Snacks

Vegetables (Target 30 per week)	Fruit (2-3 Servings per day)	Processed Foods (Avoid / Minimize)

Daily Journal / Reflection Page

Date: _____

Today I am grateful for:

- _____
- _____
- _____

Important Tasks for Today:

_____
_____
_____

One thing that made me feel proud / happy:

_____

One thing that made me stressed / challenged:

_____

Daily Reflection:

_____
_____
_____
_____
_____
_____
_____

DAILY FOOD JOURNAL

Current Weight: _____

Breakfast: _____ am

Lunch: _____ pm

Dinner _____ pm

Snacks

Vegetables (Target 30 per week)	Fruit (2-3 Servings per day)	Processed Foods (Avoid / Minimize)

Daily Journal / Reflection Page

Date: _____

Today I am grateful for:

- _____
- _____
- _____

Important Tasks for Today:

_____
_____
_____

One thing that made me feel proud / happy:

_____

One thing that made me stressed / challenged:

_____

Daily Reflection:

_____
_____
_____
_____
_____
_____
_____
_____

DAILY FOOD JOURNAL

Current Weight:

Breakfast: _____ am

Lunch: _____ pm

Dinner _____ pm

Snacks

Vegetables (Target 30 per week)	Fruit (2-3 Servings per day)	Processed Foods (Avoid / Minimize)

Daily Journal / Reflection Page

Date: _____

Today I am grateful for:

- _____
- _____
- _____

Important Tasks for Today:

_____
_____
_____

One thing that made me feel proud / happy:

_____

One thing that made me stressed / challenged:

_____

Daily Reflection:

_____
_____
_____
_____
_____
_____
_____

DAILY FOOD JOURNAL

Current Weight:

Breakfast: _____ am

Lunch: _____ pm

Dinner _____ pm

Snacks

Vegetables (Target 30 per week)	Fruit (2-3 Servings per day)	Processed Foods (Avoid / Minimize)

Deep Reflection Prompts

Use these prompts inspired by Jerry Colonna when you feel the need for deeper introspection:

- How have I been complicit in creating the condition I say I do not want?

  _____
  _____

- What am I not saying that needs to be said?

  _____
  _____

- What is being said that I am not hearing?

  _____
  _____

- Right now, I am feeling…

  _____
  _____

- In what ways do I deplete myself and run myself into the ground?

  _____
  _____

- Where am I running from and where am I running to?

  _____
  _____

Weekly Review Prompts

- What progress have I made this week on my habits?

  _____

  _____

- Where did I feel most energized?

  _____

  _____

- What challenges did I face, and how did I respond?

  _____

  _____

- What could I improve for next week?

  _____

  _____

- Which habit or mindset helped me most?

  _____

  _____

Top 3 Goals for the Coming Week:

1. _____
2. _____
3. _____

"I've learned that people will forget what you said, people will forget what you did, but people will never forget how you made them feel."

– *Maya Angelou*

Weekly Habit Tracker

Track your habits using the SHAVE GAMERS framework. Use this weekly template to keep yourself accountable:

Habits:	Monday	Tuesday	Wednesday	Thursday	Friday	Saturday	Sunday
Sleep							
Hydration							
Affirmations							
Visualizations							
Exercise							
Gratitude							
Audible / Learning							
Meditation							
Eat Healthy							
Relationships							
Scribing							

WEEKLY FITNESS TRACKER

Monday	Daily Steps:	Duration:
Workout		

Tuesday	Daily Steps:	Duration:
Workout		

Wednesday	Daily Steps:	Duration:
Workout		

Thursday	Daily Steps:	Duration:
Workout		

Friday	Daily Steps:	Duration:
Workout		

Saturday	Daily Steps:	Duration:
Workout		

Sunday	Daily Steps:	Duration:
Workout		

Daily Journal / Reflection Page

Date: _____

Today I am grateful for:

- _____
- _____
- _____

Important Tasks for Today:

_____
_____
_____

One thing that made me feel proud / happy:

_____

One thing that made me stressed / challenged:

_____

Daily Reflection:

_____
_____
_____
_____
_____
_____
_____
_____

DAILY FOOD JOURNAL

Current Weight:

Breakfast: _____am

Lunch: _____pm

Dinner _____pm

Snacks

Vegetables (Target 30 per week)	Fruit (2-3 Servings per day)	Processed Foods (Avoid / Minimize)

Daily Journal / Reflection Page

Date: _____

Today I am grateful for:

- _____
- _____
- _____

Important Tasks for Today:

_____
_____
_____

One thing that made me feel proud / happy:

_____

One thing that made me stressed / challenged:

_____

Daily Reflection:

_____
_____
_____
_____
_____
_____
_____

DAILY FOOD JOURNAL

Current Weight: _____

Breakfast: _____ am

Lunch: _____ pm

Dinner _____ pm

Snacks

Vegetables (Target 30 per week)	Fruit (2-3 Servings per day)	Processed Foods (Avoid / Minimize)

Daily Journal / Reflection Page

Date: _____

Today I am grateful for:

- _____
- _____
- _____

Important Tasks for Today:

_____
_____
_____

One thing that made me feel proud / happy:

_____

One thing that made me stressed / challenged:

_____

Daily Reflection:

_____
_____
_____
_____
_____
_____
_____

DAILY FOOD JOURNAL

Current Weight:

Breakfast: _____ am

Lunch: _____ pm

Dinner _____ pm

Snacks

Vegetables (Target 30 per week)	Fruit (2-3 Servings per day)	Processed Foods (Avoid / Minimize)

Daily Journal / Reflection Page

Date: _____

Today I am grateful for:

- _____
- _____
- _____

Important Tasks for Today:

_____
_____
_____

One thing that made me feel proud / happy:

_____

One thing that made me stressed / challenged:

_____

Daily Reflection:

_____
_____
_____
_____
_____
_____
_____

DAILY FOOD JOURNAL

Current Weight: _____

Breakfast: _____ am

Lunch: _____ pm

Dinner _____ pm

Snacks

Vegetables (Target 30 per week)	Fruit (2-3 Servings per day)	Processed Foods (Avoid / Minimize)

Daily Journal / Reflection Page

Date: _____

Today I am grateful for:

- _____
- _____
- _____

Important Tasks for Today:

_____
_____
_____

One thing that made me feel proud / happy:

_____

One thing that made me stressed / challenged:

_____

Daily Reflection:

_____
_____
_____
_____
_____
_____
_____

DAILY FOOD JOURNAL

Current Weight:

Breakfast: _____am

Lunch: _____pm

Dinner _____pm

Snacks

Vegetables (Target 30 per week)	Fruit (2-3 Servings per day)	Processed Foods (Avoid / Minimize)

Daily Journal / Reflection Page

Date: _____

Today I am grateful for:

- _____
- _____
- _____

Important Tasks for Today:

_____
_____
_____

One thing that made me feel proud / happy:

_____

One thing that made me stressed / challenged:

_____

Daily Reflection:

_____
_____
_____
_____
_____
_____
_____
_____

DAILY FOOD JOURNAL

Current Weight:

Breakfast: _____ am
Lunch: _____ pm
Dinner _____ pm
Snacks

Vegetables (Target 30 per week)	Fruit (2-3 Servings per day)	Processed Foods (Avoid / Minimize)

Daily Journal / Reflection Page

Date: _____

Today I am grateful for:

- _____
- _____
- _____

Important Tasks for Today:

_____
_____
_____

One thing that made me feel proud / happy:

_____

One thing that made me stressed / challenged:

_____

Daily Reflection:

_____
_____
_____
_____
_____
_____
_____

DAILY FOOD JOURNAL

Current Weight:

Breakfast: _____am
Lunch: _____pm
Dinner _____pm
Snacks

Vegetables (Target 30 per week)	Fruit (2-3 Servings per day)	Processed Foods (Avoid / Minimize)

Deep Reflection Prompts

Use these prompts inspired by Jerry Colonna when you feel the need for deeper introspection:

- How have I been complicit in creating the condition I say I do not want?

- What am I not saying that needs to be said?

- What is being said that I am not hearing?

- Right now, I am feeling…

- In what ways do I deplete myself and run myself into the ground?

- Where am I running from and where am I running to?

Weekly Review Prompts

- What progress have I made this week on my habits?

    _____
    _____

- Where did I feel most energized?

    _____
    _____

- What challenges did I face, and how did I respond?

    _____
    _____

- What could I improve for next week?

    _____
    _____

- Which habit or mindset helped me most?

    _____
    _____

Top 3 Goals for the Coming Week:

1. _____
2. _____
3. _____

"If everyone would sweep their own doorstep, the whole world would be clean."

– Mother Teresa

Weekly Habit Tracker

Track your habits using the **SHAVE GAMERS** framework. Use this weekly template to keep yourself accountable:

Habits:	Monday	Tuesday	Wednesday	Thursday	Friday	Saturday	Sunday
Sleep							
Hydration							
Affirmations							
Visualizations							
Exercise							
Gratitude							
Audible / Learning							
Meditation							
Eat Healthy							
Relationships							
Scribing							

WEEKLY FITNESS TRACKER

Monday	Daily Steps:	Duration:
Workout		

Tuesday	Daily Steps:	Duration:
Workout		

Wednesday	Daily Steps:	Duration:
Workout		

Thursday	Daily Steps:	Duration:
Workout		

Friday	Daily Steps:	Duration:
Workout		

Saturday	Daily Steps:	Duration:
Workout		

Sunday	Daily Steps:	Duration:
Workout		

Daily Journal / Reflection Page

Date: _____

Today I am grateful for:

- _____
- _____
- _____

Important Tasks for Today:

_____
_____
_____

One thing that made me feel proud / happy:

_____

One thing that made me stressed / challenged:

_____

Daily Reflection:

_____
_____
_____
_____
_____
_____
_____

DAILY FOOD JOURNAL

Current Weight: _____

Breakfast: _____ am
Lunch: _____ pm
Dinner _____ pm
Snacks

Vegetables (Target 30 per week)	Fruit (2-3 Servings per day)	Processed Foods (Avoid / Minimize)

Daily Journal / Reflection Page

Date: _____

Today I am grateful for:

- _____
- _____
- _____

Important Tasks for Today:

_____
_____
_____

One thing that made me feel proud / happy:

_____

One thing that made me stressed / challenged:

_____

Daily Reflection:

_____
_____
_____
_____
_____
_____
_____
_____

DAILY FOOD JOURNAL

Current Weight: _____

Breakfast: _____am
Lunch: _____pm
Dinner _____pm
Snacks

Vegetables (Target 30 per week)	Fruit (2-3 Servings per day)	Processed Foods (Avoid / Minimize)

Daily Journal / Reflection Page

Date: _____

Today I am grateful for:

- _____
- _____
- _____

Important Tasks for Today:

_____
_____
_____

One thing that made me feel proud / happy:

_____

One thing that made me stressed / challenged:

_____

Daily Reflection:

_____
_____
_____
_____
_____
_____
_____

DAILY FOOD JOURNAL

Current Weight: _____

Breakfast: _____ am
Lunch: _____ pm
Dinner _____ pm
Snacks

Vegetables (Target 30 per week)	Fruit (2-3 Servings per day)	Processed Foods (Avoid / Minimize)

Daily Journal / Reflection Page

Date: _____

Today I am grateful for:

- _____
- _____
- _____

Important Tasks for Today:

_____
_____
_____

One thing that made me feel proud / happy:

_____

One thing that made me stressed / challenged:

_____

Daily Reflection:

_____
_____
_____
_____
_____
_____
_____
_____

DAILY FOOD JOURNAL

Current Weight:

Breakfast: _____ am

Lunch: _____ pm

Dinner _____ pm

Snacks

Vegetables (Target 30 per week)	Fruit (2-3 Servings per day)	Processed Foods (Avoid / Minimize)

Daily Journal / Reflection Page

Date: _____

Today I am grateful for:

- _____
- _____
- _____

Important Tasks for Today:

_____
_____
_____

One thing that made me feel proud / happy:

_____

One thing that made me stressed / challenged:

_____

Daily Reflection:

_____
_____
_____
_____
_____
_____
_____
_____

DAILY FOOD JOURNAL

Current Weight:

Breakfast: _____ am

Lunch: _____ pm

Dinner _____ pm

Snacks

Vegetables (Target 30 per week)	Fruit (2-3 Servings per day)	Processed Foods (Avoid / Minimize)

Daily Journal / Reflection Page

Date: _____

Today I am grateful for:

- _____
- _____
- _____

Important Tasks for Today:

_____
_____
_____

One thing that made me feel proud / happy:

_____

One thing that made me stressed / challenged:

_____

Daily Reflection:

_____
_____
_____
_____
_____
_____
_____
_____

DAILY FOOD JOURNAL

Current Weight: _____

Breakfast: _____ am

Lunch: _____ pm

Dinner _____ pm

Snacks

Vegetables (Target 30 per week)	Fruit (2-3 Servings per day)	Processed Foods (Avoid / Minimize)

Daily Journal / Reflection Page

Date: _____

Today I am grateful for:

- _____
- _____
- _____

Important Tasks for Today:

_____
_____
_____
_____

One thing that made me feel proud / happy:

_____

One thing that made me stressed / challenged:

_____

Daily Reflection:

_____
_____
_____
_____
_____
_____
_____
_____

DAILY FOOD JOURNAL

Current Weight: _____

Breakfast: _____ am
Lunch: _____ pm
Dinner _____ pm
Snacks

Vegetables (Target 30 per week)	Fruit (2-3 Servings per day)	Processed Foods (Avoid / Minimize)

Deep Reflection Prompts

Use these prompts inspired by Jerry Colonna when you feel the need for deeper introspection:

- How have I been complicit in creating the condition I say I do not want?

- What am I not saying that needs to be said?

- What is being said that I am not hearing?

- Right now, I am feeling…

- In what ways do I deplete myself and run myself into the ground?

- Where am I running from and where am I running to?

Weekly Review Prompts

- What progress have I made this week on my habits?

  _____
  _____

- Where did I feel most energized?

  _____
  _____

- What challenges did I face, and how did I respond?

  _____
  _____

- What could I improve for next week?

  _____
  _____

- Which habit or mindset helped me most?

  _____
  _____

Top 3 Goals for the Coming Week:

1. _____
2. _____
3. _____

www.ingramcontent.com/pod-product-compliance
Lightning Source LLC
Chambersburg PA
CBHW080540030426
42337CB00024B/4808